BY CANDLELIGHT
candles for scent, mood, and romance

Diana Rosen

The mission of Storey Publishing is to serve our customers
by publishing practical information that encourages personal independence
in harmony with the environment.

Edited by Deborah Balmuth, Jennifer Travis Donnelly, and Carey Boucher
Cover design by Wendy Palitz
Cover illustration © Juliette Borda
Interior illustrations by Laura Tedeschi
Text design by Susan Bernier
Text production by Jennifer Jepson Smith

The information in this book is true and complete to the best of our knowledge. All recommendations are made without guarantee on the part of the author or Storey Publishing. The author and publisher disclaim any liability in connection with the use of this information. For additional information, please contact Storey Publishing, 210 MASS MoCA Way, North Adams, MA 01247.

Storey books are available for special premium and promotional uses and for customized editions. For further information, please call 1-800-793-9396.

Printed in the United States by Lake Book
10 9 8 7 6 5 4 3 2 1

ISBN 1-58017-566-X

Making "Scents" of Candlelight

Choosing scented candles to match our mood or meet our needs adds a new dimension to these ancient forms of illumination. Candles become not just a vehicle for light, but a special gift we can share at holidays and celebrations; in times of meditation or prayer; or to add a touch of the extraordinary to the everyday.

Holiday Scents

Aromatherapy is an ancient science that has defined particular scents as energizing, relaxing, stimulating, healing, or soothing. It reminds us of the power of nature's bounty to lift our spirits, treat our ills, or help us regenerate. Flowers, trees, herbs, plants, and foods not only bring healing, they open up the well of memory to bring us back to those special times in our life that we connect with particular aromas. For example, the sharp/sweet tang of orange zest, the bite of clove or ginger, and the sweet earthiness of pumpkin are signature scents of the Thanksgiving season; frankincense, myrrh, cinnamon, peppermint, and pine can remind us of the winter holidays. The endearing sweetness of rose conjures gentle thoughts of Valentine's Day, Mother's Day, or wedding anniversaries.

―――――――

The light of memory, or rather the light
that memory lends to things, is the palest light of all . . .
memory makes me profoundly aware of . . . the evanescence
of the world, a fleeting image in the moving water.

— Eugène Ionesco,
Present Past — Past Present

―――――――

Bayberry for the New Year

New Englanders have a saying that goes, *"A bayberry candle, burned to the socket, puts luck in the home, food in the larder, and gold in the pocket."* While we can't swear it's true, it's such a nice idea that we suggest providing bayberry candles as New Year's Day gifts for everyone who comes over to dine on your black-eyed peas — an absolutely, positively, no-doubt-about-it, bring-you-luck custom!

Meditation and Relaxation Scents

The power of scent is an important ingredient in the recipe for de-stressing, relaxing, meditating, or healing the hurt of separation, loss, or other grief. Scents can make the most of your meditation experience. Meditation can be casual or ritualized, but to be most effective, it does require silence and space. The addition of a candle scented with essence of jasmine, sandalwood, aloeswood, or lotus can do much to transport you to a center of calm.

*Come hither, and I shall light a candle of understanding
in thine heart, which shall not be put out.*

—Apocrypha 2, Esdras, 14–25

Pick a space that is uncluttered, away from distractions, and comfortable. Light your candle and place it nearby, but not so close that its aroma might overwhelm you. The spiritual focus of a room is often the northwest area; if you have a place for your candle there, you should use it.

Sit quietly in a chair, lay down on your bed or couch, or sit on a floor cushion.

You'll quickly discover how the scent of a candle complements the solitude and helps you dip into feelings of gratitude, love, and sweet remembrances. You will discover a depth of nurturing that will encourage you on the path to healing from your loss, relaxing from the tension of the day, or finding a clarity with which to solve the problems of the hour.

Engaging in this relaxation practice for just ten minutes is very powerful, yet if you can allow yourself twenty or thirty minutes, the effect will last longer and be stronger, enabling you to pursue your goals for the day with a new font of energy.

Energizing Scents

The familiar midmorning kaffe klatch or afternoon tea break helps us separate ourselves from the hectic pace of the day to experience the renewing comfort of a fragrant beverage drunk alone or with companions. Often, a cup of freshly brewed tea is all we need to feel energized enough to finish the day. At other times, the soothing sweetness of hot chocolate or the richness of a coffee drink is pure satisfaction. Yet, there may be days when you need not refreshment for your body but the regeneration that comes only from the solace of solitude.

The Candle Energizing Break, described below, can help you fill this need. Aromatherapy suggests using a candle imbued with the energizing power of ginger, clove, verbena, lemon balm, grapefruit, orange, or lime.

No matter where you are, find a place where you can shut the door. Pull your shoes off, dim the lights, and turn off any noisy equipment (especially the telephone!). Place the candle in the northeast section of the room, which many consider to represent self-knowledge, and light it.

* Be still.
* Breathe.
* Close your eyes and rest.
* Stretch gently.
* Walk around the room several times, slowly, as if you were walking a labyrinth.
* Sit down and inhale the fresh smell of your candle.
* Close your eyes again and rest.

✳ When you feel the last of the tension escape your body, stand up again and stretch once more. You'll feel a keen sense of clarity and energy that will take you through rest of the day with happy resolve.

✳ Extinguish the candle; repeat on another day.

Celebrating with Candlelight

... the marvelous loveliness of light ...
— St. Augustine, *City of God*

Entertaining friends and family on a Sunday afternoon or at a holiday dinner calls for candles! Candlelight sets the mood, enhances the festivities, and adds a feeling of welcoming hospitality to any gathering.

Yes, you can bring out your favorite candlesticks and tapers; they're an elegant and traditional way to accent a dining or buffet table. And yes, bring out your "good" candlesticks; never wait for special occasions. Today is the best time to enjoy your treasures. However, if you're searching for more creative effects, here are some other ideas to add a sparkling highlight to your home entertaining.

Candle Centerpiece. Instead of the bowl of fruit or vase of flowers at the center of the table, make a centerpiece of candles! Place a large group of candlesticks of all heights together atop a group of trivets or heat-resistant tiles. If you need "height," place a few candles on a pedestal cake dish.

Gather together all of the brass candlesticks, or all of the silver ones, or mix them up; have fun!

Tip: When adding candles to a buffet table, use only unscented or beeswax candles, which do not "fight" the inviting aroma of food.

Mirrors Reflect Light. Place a mirror face-up on your table. On its surface, line up a row of clear glass votives containing white candles. The combination of silvery mirror, clear glass, and pure white makes this centerpiece a sparkling vision. For an extra touch, weave curlicues of satin ribbon back and forth between the votives. Follow the white and silver theme, or add your favorite pastels or vibrant hues.

Floating Candles. Floating candles are intriguing and, yes, they do float! These flat-bottomed candles come in shapes of stars, flowers, ovals, or rounds and in an assortment of colors. As a happy surprise for your guests, place them in a cut-glass or translucent, colored glass bowl of water, and light them just before the guests arrive at the table. For additional glamour, add one gorgeous lotus flower in the center of the bowl.

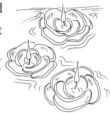

Gourds for Candlesticks. The jack o'lantern with its interior candle projecting light through a scary face is a highlight of Halloween, and the choice of styles and shapes of pumpkins is amazing. Most delightful for candle lovers are the miniature pumpkins and small gourds that your grocer offers in the fall. They make marvelous candle holders.

Carve out and discard the stems of gourds, pumpkins, or apples. Deepen the holes as needed so that tapers stand upright. If the gourd is wobbly, slice off the bottom so it stands straight. Put in tapers and arrange the gourds on a cookie sheet lined with colorful fall leaves soaked in water. Light the candles for the most creative centerpiece ever!

Candelabra. Hosting an elegant candlelight tea? Toasting the New Year with a midnight ball? Splurge with a silver candelabra! Find the most elaborate one the party rental company has to offer and bring it to the party. Add sparkle-dusted tapers and encircle the candelabra with strings of silvery ribbon and small white votive candles in silvertone holders. The result? Total drama, glamour, and excitement for you and your guests.

Any Wednesday

Why wait for holidays or special events to light candles for dinner? Wednesday is as good a reason as any! Whether you have one child or ten, whether dinner is a pepperoni pizza and salad or a full roast-chicken dinner with all the side dishes, bring out some candles.

For a pizza party, duplicate what the Italian restaurants do. Bring out that checkered tablecloth from the picnic basket, put the pizza on a pedestal stand, stick a candle in an old wine or olive oil bottle, light it, and then turn off the lights.

Planning a more elaborate meal? Bring our your prettiest table linens, your best dinnerware and cutlery, and the nicest candlesticks. Arrange the food on the table, light the candles, and turn off the electric lights.

Then, call everyone to the table, and watch their faces! There's something about candlelight that says "you're special" to everyone at the table whether you're serving pizza, leftovers, or a full-course meal.

Candlelight creates a gentle, subdued atmosphere that encourages everyone to eat slowly, talk quietly, and fully relax. Wednesdays will never be ordinary again!

Smell is a potent wizard that transports us across thousands of miles and all the years we've loved.
— Helen Keller

Candlelight Isn't Just for Dinner

Winter Mornings. Wintertime mornings are rough if you live in a cold climate. The warmth of hot oatmeal and cocoa can go a long way to getting a good start on the day, but next time you're faced with the gray of a blustery morning, why not have breakfast by candlelight? It's a soft way to ease into the day feeling nourished with good food and blessed with those who share your home.

Summer Picnics. For a summertime candleholder, turn over a carved-out half of a watermelon rind. Cut a few holes in the rind that are big enough for tapers, and voila! You have an amusing, biodegradable centerpiece. Light the candles as twilight falls, and settle down to listen to tall tales, stories about your ancestors from visiting relatives, or just the cricket symphony playing as the stars make their entrance in the dark of the sky.

Afternoon Tea. At any time of the year, afternoon tea is tailor-made for the relaxation of being with friends. Add to the softness of the time with carefully placed candles on your serving tray or on flat surfaces near where you and your friends gather. The sun's still shining? No matter, candles will still enchant and delight, just because they'll be unexpected.

What's a Birthday Without Candles?

Children's Birthdays. Birthday candles aren't simply white anymore; they come in many colors, stripes, and patterns. The tradition is to decorate a cake with a number of candles equal to the age of the birthday boy or girl. This year, mix up colors and patterns for a riot of color, or spell out the child's age instead of placing a certain number of candles here and there. For example, for a ten-year-old, make a one and a zero out of big candles in your child's favorite colors or happy stripes or fun circles. If the child has a short name, spell it out with candles.

If a cartoon character or particular animal is your child's delight, seek out one fat candle shaped like her favorite and light it as a solitary birthday candle. Or give lots of these candles to the party guests as favors, keeping several more for the party honoree, of course!

Adult Birthdays. For those of us considerably older than ten, forty or fifty or more candles on a cake might look more like a campfire than a celebration. Here's a stunning way to celebrate an adult birthday in an unconventional way, especially for small groups of six to eight guests.

Ask a guest to whisk away the honoree while you place a small matchbox and a red candle in a beribboned votive holder in front of each place setting. Ask the guests to light their candles before you turn out the electric lights. Your birthday honoree will certainly be expecting a cake with candles but will be unprepared to see an elegant array of small beautiful red candles shining brightly around the table in front of the guests standing to greet him or her.

Instead of boisterous singing, the guests can make a wish for the birthday celebrant's upcoming year, either funny or serious. After revealing the wish, the guest blows out his or her candle. When the last candle is extinguished, you can turn the lights back on and everyone can sing "Happy Birthday" as a prelude to generous slices of a yummy birthday cake.

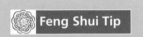

Feng Shui Tip

Whether indoors or out-doors, avoid placing can-dles in the west or northwest areas of the house or garden. Feng shui experts believe that these areas are "metal" areas, and fire can melt them or eliminate the strength of these places.

Candlelight Outdoors

When you are entertaining outside, candles can set the mood and, in humid places, repel bothersome mosquitoes. Citronella, which has a delectable lemony smell to us humans, is unpleasant to mosquitoes, so add citronella candles lavishly around your patio or garden.

You can welcome guests with a row of luminaria along the path to your door. Luminaria are paper bags, filled with sand, that do double duty: The sand holds the bags steadily in place, and they also safely hold small votive holders containing lit candles. The candlelight will shine through even a Kraft bag, but you might want to cut out little diamond shapes or criss-cross marks to emit even more light.

Many patio furniture shops and catalogs sell lantern poles that can be stuck firmly into the ground around your garden. The lanterns are suitable both for illumination and as a container for citronella candles to repel insects.

For dinner for two on the balcony, candles are a must. Short ones are great, or add a clear glass lantern cover for tapers to protect yourself and your beautiful dinner table from breezes that could extinguish the flame or topple a candlestick.

Note: When using candles out of doors, keep a pail of water nearby, "just in case," especially if you have no water hose. Save the fire extinguisher for indoors.

Smells are surer than sounds and sights
to make heartstrings crack

— Rudyard Kipling

Honoring Traditions
and Memories

All of us stage "altars" about our homes to remind us of the people, places, and things that give us pleasure. One of the most familiar altars is a loving collection of family photos set upon a fireplace mantel, grouped together on a table, or hung along a wall.

Placing candlelight near these precious photographs casts soft light on our favorite faces. Set a votive candle in front of several different photos, or place a larger candle on a pedestal and stand the photos in a circle around the candle. Or set the revered photos atop a pedestal and light the images from below with a candle.

Memory Candle

Lighting candles is a timeless way to honor the memory of loved ones who have passed on. One way to invoke someone's memory is to make a Memory Candle by taping a pretty piece of paper imprinted with the person's image around a clear glass candle holder. It's simple to do.

1. Select a photo and a clear glass candle holder.

2. Measure the height of the candle holder, top to bottom.

3. Make a copy of the photo onto a piece of parchment-like paper, available in many colors at your local copy shop. Reduce or enlarge the photo to match the height of the holder.

4. Cut the paper to size and wrap it around the outside of the holder, taping it securely.

5. Light the candle inside the votive. The soft glow of candlelight will illuminate the "photograph" in a very special way.

This commemorative candle can also acknowledge a well-loved pet or the memory of an important person in your community.

Honor Candle

You can also pay homage to the living by naming this an "honor candle" and using a photograph to celebrate a graduation, marriage, birth, retirement, anniversary, or any accomplishment of note.

Pampering Yourself
with Candlelight

Reading by candlelight may seem quaint, yet even the most difficult textbook seems easier to digest when a group of candles illuminates its pages. Certainly, reading a treasured novel or beloved poem could not be more enjoyable than by candlelight. And reading poetry by candlelight to your mate is sublime!

Your candlestick or votive holder should blend in well with your desk and accessories, and it should be as important a home accessory as a pillow or a picture frame. Brass is lovely with wood; silver goes with everything; and with wood, painted or plain porcelain, and clear cut glass, the choices for candlesticks are breathtaking. You can purchase colorful ones from Africa, Central and South America, India, or Morocco. Pick one or several; group them or spread them around you; put some high up on shelves and others at desk level or beside your chair. Make these "your candlesticks," to be used only by you in your special corner.

Candles should heighten the pleasure of reading or listening to music. If it's the light of the candles that soothes you, plain unscented candles or gentle beeswax candles with their delicate honey smell will work very well. If you want a full sensory experience, spicy or citrus scents are stimulating for studying, and florals are lovely for listening to music.

If you want to enhance your studies, blue, turquoise, or green candles are very powerful. These should be positioned in the northeast part of the room, even if that means they're far away from your desk. You can light others at your desk for light and comfort, but the best place for a desk is the northeast area of a room, which is the area representing knowledge.

Now, settle into your chair, put on that CD or gather your books around you, light the candle, and dive into the pleasures of music and reading, surrounded by the shimmering glow of candlelight.

Bathing by Candlelight

Ah, the absolute luxury of a warm bath; is there a better gift to yourself than time in the tub? It's so important, it may even be worth it to trade babysitting hours with a friend, have a noontime experience while the kids are in school, or bathe while they nap. Whatever you can do to squeeze in this experience, do it! You'll be so glad you did.

A great bathing experience requires a plan. First, make arrangements to have the bathroom all to yourself. Post a "DO NOT DISTURB" sign on the door, if necessary. Your family will soon get the idea that this is your private time.

Beauty sat bathing by a spring . . .
— Anthony Munday
"Primaleon of Greece"

Now, for the pleasures:

* Choose the biggest, fluffiest towels you have in the closet.

* Bring in your favorite soaps, bubble baths, and oils.

* Match candles to the scents of your soaps or use candles that are unscented. Place them away from fabric. If possible, one candle should be reflected by mirrors.

* Light the candles.

* Turn on the water full force and watch the bubbles explode or the oils swirl in the water.

* Switch off the lights, step carefully into the tub, sit down, lean back, close your eyes, and enjoy, enjoy, enjoy. Silence. Sweet smells. Warm water. Hmmm . . . .

More of a Good Thing!

"Clean fun" takes on a whole new meaning when you share a tub with someone you love. Bubbles aren't just for women; men love the delight they bring. And what's nicer than having someone right there to wash your back?

Sharing the pleasure of the bath demands the sensual pleasure of soft candlelight with the romantic touch of vanilla, ylang-ylang, or rose. Again, pile soft, fresh towels onto the counter, open up new soaps, light the candles, flip off the lights, and sink into the tub with you-know-who. You can take it from here . . .

A New Twist on Bathing the Kids

Nighttime bathing is a ritual for some families. The children can unwind with rubber toys while mom or dad helps wash the dirt of the day from little toes and noses. You can add the calming presence of candlelight to make something extraordinary out of the daily bath.

As the kids bathe, dim the lights and set a lit candle near a mirror to add the mysterious softness to the room. Sit on the edge of the tub (or wherever is most comfortable) and read a "bathtime story." As the kids towel off and don their jammies, the novelty of the evening is bound to give them sweet dreams that will come before their heads touch the pillows.

How many miles to Babylon?
Three score and ten.
Can I get there by candlelight?
Yes, and back again.

— Mother Goose

The Bedroom

Candles imbued with lavender are the ultimate sleep aid! Women, for centuries, have added the clean fresh fragrance of lavender to rinse water for laundering bed sheets, and they have slipped in dried lavender flowers to impart a delicate perfume to lingerie drawers or dream pillows. Light your lavender fragranced candle tonight as you prepare for bed; its light, lovely aroma will surely bring you delicious dreams. Just be sure to extinguish it before you fall asleep.

Candles of rose, vanilla, or jasmine are wonderful for the bedroom. Their fragrance brings relaxation and calm, and their flaming light brings a peace and quiet nothing else quite matches.

Throughout the year, mark each solstice with a special lighting of cleansing lavender, pine, or citrus candles. Mark these full-moon nights: March 21, June 21, September 21, and December 21. Open up the windows afterward to allow any and all negative energy to whisk away, leaving your bedroom fresh and blessed.

Soft, soft I have made my bed . . . Come, let us lose ourselves in dalliance, all the night through, let us enjoy the long-desired embrace . . .

—Proverbs 7:16–18

Love Candles

Love inflames the heart! And nothing complements love better than a burning candle softly casting its bright golden glow upon the framed photograph of your beloved. Candles are a natural part of creating the delightful romance that can help keep you two together. But what if you don't have someone significant in your life? What can candles do for you? A Love Candle could very well be the light that brings a lover to you!

A Love Candle is made in the same way as a Memory Candle (see page 22) except that it has a wish list wrapped around it instead of an image of a friend or loved one.

Here's how easy it is to do:

1. Buy some pretty paper, preferably pink or peach, that will allow light to shine through it. Tissue and parchment paper both work well.

2. With a calligraphy pen of black ink or a traditional pen with purple or red ink, write down on the paper all the

qualities you seek in a lover. Be very specific. Choose your words carefully, because you may get what you wish for! Some words to include are kind, fun, funny, tall, short, religious, smart, generous, loves children, good with pets, good cook (we can ask!), affectionate, adventurous, brave, or any other quality your heart desires.

3. Select a clear glass holder for any kind of candle you like, although vanilla, rose, and ylang-ylang are timeless fragrances of love. Special colors for love are pink, red, orange, yellow, or white, but peach is the ultimate for the unmarried.

4. Tape the paper firmly around the candle holder.

5. Light the candle only when you are alone, repeat out loud the words you've written, and allow the candle to burn completely.

6. Repeat as often as you like!

Note: If possible, place your Love Candle in the southwest area of your bedroom. This is the area of marriage, romance and love. Peonies are said to draw the ideal mate to an unmarried girl. Position a bouquet of peonies, or a photograph of one, next to your Love Candle. Scatter some heart-shaped candles around for an extra added touch.

I love thee to the level of everyday's [sic]
Most quiet need, by sun and candle-light . . .

—Elizabeth Barrett Browning,
"How Do I Love Thee?"
from *Sonnets of the Portuguese*

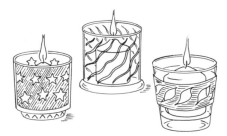

Candles:
Everyone's Favorite Gift!

Nothing is easier to give, or nicer to receive, than candles. They come in all sizes and shapes, unscented or scented, and you can suit everyone on your gift list with the totally practical, the whimsical or irreverent, the elegant or serene, the purest soy candle or the most outrageously tacky sparkle-encrusted towering taper.

Beeswax or unscented candles are best for anyone whose fragrance favorites you don't know. Both come in endless sizes and shapes, and their neutral white or honey colors take to any color ribbon, fabric, or gift bag.

Votive holders are another "generic" gift for the candle lover. Even the plainest clear holder can be decorated with fun or elegant stickers or ribbons and bows, or set into tiny tin pails or terra cotta flower pots with a piece of foil covering up the drainage hole. (The pails and pots are terrific party favors, too!)

Bobeches

If you have absolute traditionalists on your gift list, consider a set of glass bobeches (wax shields). These glass discs have a hole in the middle so that you can slip them over a taper and rest them on the lip of a candlestick. They catch the drips of candle wax, preventing them from falling onto fine linens or the candlestick itself. They come etched, curved, plain, or patterned and are available wherever fine dining accessories are sold.

Candle Snuffers

Candle snuffers offer clever choices in styles and designs. And their function is complemented by their beauty. Highly collectible (they've been manufactured for centuries), candle snuffers can be very plain or elaborately decorated with the most fanciful ornamentation in brass, silver, tin, or iron. Prior to the late 19th century, snuffers were called *douters*, because they "do out" a flame. Many antique and most modern snuffers have a bell-like shape on one end of a ten- to twelve-inch handle. The bell is gently lowered over the candle's flame, thoroughly extinguishing it in a simple and safe manner.

Before 1850, the primary function of candle snuffers was not to extinguish the flame but to trim wicks and discard ash. The flame was left to burn for light in an era when creating fire was still a challenge. Matches had been invented in 1827, but it was quite a while before they became economical and easily accessible.

Creative Candle Holders

You probably have lots of candle holders around the house you didn't know you had! Here are some that are fun or practical and certainly unusual.

Round Cookie Tins or Old Metal Lunchboxes. These allow you to cram in lots of votives to make a spectacular centerpiece. If you don't have votive holders, pour some colorful pink or green lentils, or a mix of black and white beans, onto the bottoms of the tins and set the candles among them. Or, grab some sand, dirt, or pebbles from the yard for an "earthy" natural look for your centerpiece.

"Divorced" Crockery and Napkin Rings. Saucerless teacups make great votive holders, and cupless saucers are great dripping plates. Mix and match is definitely the design element here.

Etched glass plates, picture frames with glass interiors, and "lone" plates that never seem to go with anything make elegant trays for candle centerpieces. Even washed tuna or catfish tins covered in foil or painted make perfect settings for a candle.

Brass, silver, or other metal napkin rings look great on "cupless saucers" and accommodate votive candles or tea lights easily.

Leftover copper tubing from plumbing jobs also makes elegant candle holders (and napkin rings, too.)

Bottles and Jars. Narrow-necked glass bottles are great for tapers, and wide-mouth jars are clearly a match for votive candles. Just fill them with beans or lentils or, for a dash of color, toss in a few multicolored marbles or sand of different hues, and you have a charming and unique holder. Tie ribbons around the necks of the jars for added color.

Pans. Metal cupcake pans make whimsical or elegant holders for candles, and pie plates and pie pans are great for a collection of candles of all types.

Stack two or three foil mini-loaf pans together, spread clear marbles or white beans on the bottoms, and place some candles among the beans. If you're particularly ambitious, you can paint the tins, or stick silvery bows at each end.

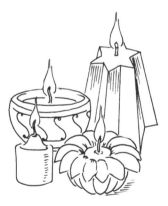

A Little History,
A Little Trivia

First came fire — roots and twigs and logs rubbed together, or two flints of rock struck against one another until sparks appeared. Fire brought warmth, a way to prepare foods previously inedible without "cooking," and a way to illuminate the dark of night both as signal and as a source of comfort.

Next came torches. Flammable resins, pitch, or natural oils were soaked into paper, papyrus, flax, or other fibers, then lit to provide bright huge flames. Torches were used to mark off boundaries, lead people through the dark, and warn or signal danger.

In our own Pacific Northwest, torches were often made of stormy petrels and "candlefish." Wicks were threaded through the cavity of the fish, and the fish was then speared with a stick that was plunged into the ground before the wick was lighted. The natural oiliness of the fish helped to keep the wick aflame.

As humans progressed in their remarkable path of trial and error, they discovered that plants, trees, insects, and animals could provide the fat or wax that could surround flammable fibers to make light in the darkness.

What Are Candles Made Of?

Ever since candle making began, beeswax and wax from vegetation have been the most common sources of candlewax. Both are having a resurgence today because of a return to the use of more natural ingredients in everything we bring into the home.

Candle makers (chandlers) in times gone by often used plant and tree materials, such as bayberries, candelilla leaves, candletree bark, esparto grass, or palm leaf varietals (carnauba and ouricury). Or they used animal byproducts, like whale oil (spermaceti), ambergris (from deer), and secretions from insects.

Stearin Solidifies

Until the 19th century, candles were often smoky and unpleasant smelling, especially those made from the fats of sheep, cows, or pigs.

In 1850, a new technique revolutionized candle making by combining paraffin with stearin, a mixture of alkali and sulfuric acid that produces a harder, longer-burning candle. To this revolutionary recipe was added palm or vegetable oils that greatly improved the strong smells once associated with candles. Stearin hardened the paraffin, the paraffin burned cleaner than previous materials, and the vegetable oils eliminated the nasty odor of animal fats.

Today, we not only have paraffin waxes, made from a petroleum base, but waxes made from vegetable or soy. Vegetable and soy waxes burn efficiently, are cleaner than paraffin, and rarely cause any allergic reactions. They also, unlike paraffin waxes, do not give off soot or airborne debris.

Gels are the newest addition to the candle family and are made not of wax, but a form of mineral oil and a polymer that helps to solidify it enough to burn. Gels can absorb more fragrance than candles.

Wick Improvements Brighten

New technology has also affected the efficacy of wicks. By braiding the fibers, chandlers made wicks that were stronger, held their position in the candle better, and burned more predictably. The fibers were treated (mordanted or pickled) to eliminate the need for constant trimming of the wick. The new wicks could burn longer and more efficiently because chemical treatments and braiding allowed the wicks to burn away from the candle and drop ashes away from the candle. This was possible because the wicks were, in fact, less flammable. Wicks are the core of a candle and make it "burn," but untreated wicks flame wildly, spew sparks, and become dangerous to everything around them.

Recent improvements in wick technology have eliminated lead as a mordant, yet these candles burn cleaner and more efficiently than ever before. Lead is no longer an acceptable part of wicking, so if you suspect that a wick contains lead, rub it lightly on a piece of paper. If the wick leaves a pencil-like mark and you are sensitive to lead, do not use that candle. Lead in wicks is illegal in the United States, but some imported candles still have wicks with lead mordants.

Along Came Electricity

Despite the improvements in wicks, waxes, and candle manufacturing, candles fell out of favor when kerosene, a steady replacement for whale oil, became the lighting source for lamps. They became even less popular when electricity was introduced in the late 19th century. Today, candles are no longer the necessity they once were for light in the darkness or for illumination for chores, reading, and other indoor activities. Instead, candles are an important part of religious ceremonies and spiritual gatherings and are revered for the charm they bring to dining and romance. However . . . when batteries die in the flashlight or when electricity falters . . . candles always come to the rescue.

What's the Difference Between a Chandelier and a Chandler?

A person who makes candles is a chandler, and the craft has been around since the 12th century. Long ago, chandlers were often divided into trade guilds of wax chandlers and tallow chandlers.

A chandelier is a hanging lamp, lit with candles or electric lights. Chandeliers are often elaborate and pretty and are frequently hung with crystal or glass beads to reflect the light of the flames or bulbs.

What's the Difference Between a Candle and a Lamp?

A candle is made from a fatty material that remains solid at room temperature, although it may melt when burned. The fatty materials might be tallow (from animal fat) or wax (beeswax or wax made from vegetables). A lamp contains fuel that is liquid at room temperature, such as oil or kerosene.

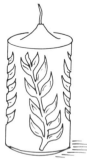

Candle Types:
Something for Everyone!

Hundreds of different kinds of candles are available today. Some of the most commonly used are described below.

Novelty: Total whimsy! These are candles molded into shapes resembling people, places, plants, flowers, animals, food, holiday symbols, cartoon characters, and anything else that the imagination can invent. These are an absolute delight to give and receive.

Pillars: These candles are defined by their thickness: two or three inches in diameter, and sometimes quite a lot more. They are usually three to six inches high, but some are gigantic. Usually round, they can also be square, hexagonal, or oval. Available scented and unscented.

Tapers: Cylindrical candles, usually six to twelve inches in height and usually ½" to ⅞" in diameter at the base. Available scented and unscented.

Tea lights. About ½" in height and the heat source for most warming pots. They easily fit into most votive holders, but they burn for only about one-third the time of a votive candle. This makes them ideal for pre-sleep time when you want only a brief candlelight experience. Available scented and unscented.

Votives: Most commonly found in areas of churches set aside for candles lit for prayers, votives have become one of the most popular types of candles for all uses. Most are short and squat, about two or three inches high and about 1½" in diameter. Available scented and unscented.

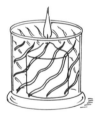

Candlemaking Methods

Like any other handmade product, candles that are hand-made include high-grade or special ingredients. They may cost a little more, but their pleasures last for hours, making them a wise investment.

Pure essential oils are more appealing than synthetic oils or scents; vegetable- and soy-based waxes are cleaner than paraffin; and the pure sweet elegance of beeswax remains the most unobtrusive yet beguiling choice for candles.

Among the many words or descriptions you'll read on packaged commercially made candles are the following.

Cast and molded: This method uses metal, cardboard, sand, or plastic molds to "case" a shape of wax that is poured into these forms.

Dipped or hand dipped: Tapers are the usual result of this method, which involves repeated dipping of a wick into melted wax. Usually a wick is draped over a short dowel and dipped into a vat of wax until enough wax has formed to make a

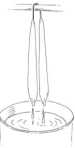

taper. A taper is narrower at the top than at the bottom, a natural result of the dipping method.

Drawn: This is a method for making birthday candles or other small narrow candles. It involves long lengths of wick, sometimes thousands of yards, that are pulled through melted wax. The wick is allowed to cool and is cut into the desired lengths.

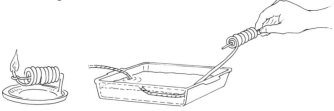

Extruded: Just like machine-made pasta, machine-made wax is extruded when wax is pushed through a shaped form (like a cookie gun). The shaped wax is then cut to the desired length.

Pressed: In this commercial method, wax is atomized onto a cooling drum, forming wax beads or granules. The beads are then compressed into molds, where they bind together and form a candle. This method is fast and produces uniform candles.

Rolled: Tapers, pillars, and some novelty candles can be made with this method, in which sheets of wax are rolled around a wick, much like pastry is rolled around a line of jelly.

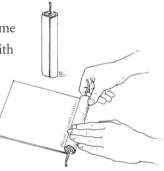

Safety Tips

1. Never leave a burning candle unattended. Never.

2. Always extinguish candles **before** going to sleep.

3. Do not place a candle close to clothes, draperies, upholstered furnishings, or other fabrics.

4. When using candles on table linens, add a bobeche (wax shield) at the base of the candle to catch drips, or place candlesticks, votives, or bare candles onto items not made of wood or fabric. Good choices are mirrors, glass, and plates.

5. If wax does drip onto linens, allow it to cool and harden, and then scrape off for easy removal.

6. Always keep candles out of reach of small children and pets.

7. Large candles should be extinguished before three hours; burning them longer may cause changes to the makeup of the wax and interfere with subsequent burning.

8. Extinguish candles by using a candle snuffer or wet paper towel placed carefully over the burning wick. Avoid blowing out a candle; a spark can fly off and onto flammable items.

9. Do not place candles in a draft. Doing so will cause excess dripping and may also blow sparks onto flammable items.

Invention of the Match

The match used to light gas stoves or candles is so common, it's hard to realize it has been around only since 1827! Previously, one needed tinder, steel, or a hardy piece of flint to light a flame.

Today there are two kinds of matches, both developed in the 1800s: the safety match, invented in 1855 by Johan Lundstrom of Sweden, and the friction match, developed in 1827 by chemist John Walker of Great Britain.

Friction matches have some form of phosphorus sulfide in the match head. This substance decomposes and burns at the low temperatures generated by friction and sets fire to the rest of the match.

What makes the safety match safe is the separation of the combustible ingredients into the match head and the striking surface on the matchbook (a mix of powdered glass, red phosphorus, and glue). You strike the match, and the friction converts the red phosphorus to white phosphorus that ignites spontaneously on contact with air (oxygen).

The match tip contains a reactive mixture of antimony trisulphide and potassium chlorate, held together by glue. Oxygen feeds the combustion elements to beget instant fire. The safety match can be struck only on the side of the box, and the friction match can be struck on anything from sandpaper to bricks.

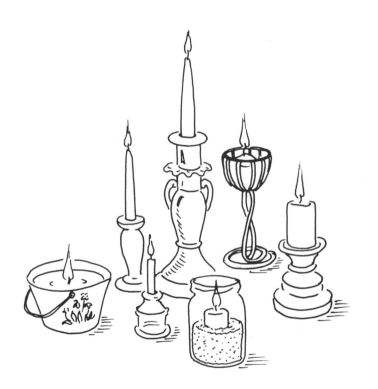

Other Storey Titles You Will Enjoy

The Candlemaker's Companion, by Betty Oppenheimer. Illustrated instructions show you how to create rolled, poured, molded, and dipped candles; add natural scent, color, and decorations; use overdipping, painting, layering, and sculpting; and create luminaria, lanterns, and floating candles. 208 pages. Paperback. ISBN 1-58017-366-7.

Gel Candles, by C. Kaila Westerman. Learn the basics of gel candle crafting in ten easy steps, and then discover how to create a wide variety of special effects with layers of color, swirls, bubbles, specialty molds, and embeddables such as glass, shells, and stones. 144 pages. Paperback. ISBN 1-58017-390-X.

Lift Me Up/Calm Me Down, by Stephanie Tourles and Barbara L. Heller. This playful, inspiring "2-books-in-1" offers dozens of great ideas, reassuring quotes, and simple suggestions for pampering yourself, whether your frazzled nerves need calming or your tired soul needs uplifting. 480 pages. Paperback. ISBN 1-58017-163-X.

These and other Storey books are available wherever books are sold and directly from Storey Publishing, 210 MASS MoCA Way, North Adams, MA 01247, or by calling 1-800-441-5700. Or visit our Web site at www.storey.com.